Unlocking the Secrets of Optimal Health

Thomas Harvey

Table of Contents

Introduction:
"Unlocking the Secrets of Optimal Health"

Welcome to the exciting journey of unlocking the secrets of optimal health. In a world where fad diets and quick fixes dominate, it's easy to get lost in the overload of conflicting information about health and wellness. But here's the truth: achieving optimal health is not a one-size-fits-all solution. It's about understanding and nurturing the unique connection between our mind, body, and soul.

In this book, we will dive deep into the core elements of optimal health, revealing the hidden secrets that have the power to transform your well-being. From the vital role of nutrition and exercise to the lesser-known factors of sleep, stress management, and social connections, we will explore various facets of health and how they are interconnected. We will also uncover the power of alternative and holistic medicine, the impact of positive emotions, and the importance of personal growth and development.

But this is not just a book of information, it is a call to action. Throughout these pages, you will discover practical tools and strategies to apply these concepts to your own life. You will learn how to tap into your inner potential, embrace a sustainable and fulfilling lifestyle, and thrive in all aspects of your well-being.

So, are you ready to uncover the secrets of optimal health and unlock a healthier, happier version of yourself? Let's embark on this journey together and discover the true potential of your mind, body, and soul. Let's begin the transformation and unlock a life of optimal health.

Chapter 1
The Mind-Body Connection: How Our Thoughts and Emotions Affect Our Health

Introduction:

The mind and body are inextricably linked, constantly interacting with and influencing each other. Our thoughts, emotions, and beliefs have a direct impact on our physical health and well-being. This connection between the mind and body has been recognized for centuries by ancient healing traditions such as Ayurveda, Traditional Chinese Medicine, and Native American medicine. More recently, modern science has also started to uncover the powerful effects of our thoughts and emotions on our physical health. In this chapter, we will explore the mind-body connection and how we can use it to improve our overall health and well-being.

The Power of Thoughts:

Thoughts are powerful. They are the driving force behind our actions and behaviors. Every thought we have creates a chemical reaction in our brain, which then sends signals to different parts of our body. Positive thoughts release feel-good hormones like dopamine and serotonin, while negative thoughts trigger stress hormones like cortisol and adrenaline.

These hormones can have a significant impact on our physical health. For instance, chronic stress, caused by negative thinking, can weaken our immune system and increase our risk of developing various health issues such as heart disease, diabetes, and depression. On the other hand, positive thoughts can boost our immune system, improve our mood, and help us cope with stress.

The Influence of Emotions:

Our emotions are closely tied to our thoughts and can also impact our physical health. Suppressing or bottling up our emotions can lead to physical tension, headaches, and digestive issues. On the other hand, expressing and processing our emotions can help us release tension and stress and promote relaxation. Studies have shown that individuals who are able to express their emotions in a healthy way have a lower risk of developing chronic health conditions.

The Mind-Body Connection in Action:

The mind-body connection is evident in many areas of our health, including pain management, immunity, and even disease prevention. For instance, research has shown that practicing mindfulness meditation, which focuses on the connection between the mind and body, can be effective in reducing chronic pain and improving overall physical and mental well-being. The mind-body connection is also crucial in strengthening our immune system. A study has found that individuals who practice positive self-talk and affirmations have a stronger immune response to flu vaccines. Furthermore, research has shown that individuals with a positive outlook on life have a lower risk of developing chronic health conditions such as heart disease and stroke.

Applying the Mind-Body Connection for Better Health:

The mind-body connection offers a powerful tool for improving our overall health and well-being. By becoming more aware of our thoughts and emotions, we can learn to manage them more effectively and experience better health outcomes. Here are a few ways we can apply the mind-body connection for better health:

1. Practice mindfulness: Mindfulness is the practice of being fully present and aware of our thoughts and surroundings. By practicing mindfulness, we can become more aware of negative thought patterns and learn to replace them with positive ones.

2. Use positive self-talk: Our internal dialogue has a significant impact on our mood and emotions. Using positive self-talk and affirmations can help us cultivate a more optimistic and resilient mindset.

3. Engage in stress-reducing activities: Chronic stress can have a detrimental effect on our physical health. Engaging in activities such as yoga, meditation, or spending time in nature can help reduce stress and promote relaxation.

4. Express and process emotions: It is essential to acknowledge and express our emotions in a healthy way. This could include talking to a trusted friend or therapist, journaling, or engaging in creative activities.

Conclusion:

The mind-body connection is a powerful tool that can significantly impact our physical health and well-being. By understanding and utilizing this connection, we can improve our overall health and prevent the development of chronic diseases. Practicing mindfulness, using positive self-talk, engaging in stress-reducing activities, and expressing and processing our emotions are all ways we can harness the power of the mind-body connection for better health. Remember, our thoughts and emotions are within our control, and by taking care of our mental health, we can see positive changes in our physical health as well.

Chapter 2: Nourishing from Within: Understanding the Importance of Nutrition

In today's fast-paced world, we often overlook the importance of nutrition in our lives. We are constantly bombarded with advertisements promoting quick and easy meals, artificial supplements, and crash diets, leaving us confused and misinformed about what healthy eating truly means. However, the truth is that proper nourishment from within is crucial for our overall well-being, both physically and mentally.

Nutrition is the process by which our body obtains and uses the necessary nutrients for growth, maintenance, and repair. These nutrients include carbohydrates, proteins, fats, vitamins, minerals, and water, and each one plays a vital role in keeping our body functioning at its best. Without a proper balance of these nutrients, our body can suffer from various health issues, affecting every aspect of our life.

One of the most significant benefits of proper nutrition is its impact on our immune system. A strong immune system is essential for fighting off diseases and infections, especially in today's world where we are constantly exposed to environmental pollutants and stressors. A diet rich in vitamins, minerals, and antioxidants can boost our immune system and help prevent illnesses.

Moreover, nutrition also plays a crucial role in maintaining a healthy weight. With the rise of obesity and related health problems, it is essential to understand the importance of a balanced diet in maintaining a healthy weight. Consuming excess calories, especially from unhealthy sources such as processed and sugary foods, can lead to weight gain and increase the risk of chronic illnesses such as diabetes, heart disease, and certain types of cancers.

In addition to physical health, proper nutrition also has a significant impact on our mental health and well-being. Studies have shown that a healthy diet can improve mood, increase energy levels, and reduce symptoms of anxiety and depression. On the other hand, a diet lacking in essential nutrients can lead to fatigue, irritability, and cognitive impairment.

Furthermore, understanding the importance of nutrition can also aid in disease prevention and management. Certain conditions, such as diabetes and heart disease, can be managed better with a balanced and nutritious diet. In some cases, a proper diet can also help reverse the effects of these chronic diseases.

It is essential to note that proper nutrition does not mean restrictive diets or depriving ourselves of our favorite foods. It is about making informed and mindful choices about what we put into our bodies. It is about incorporating a variety of whole, unprocessed foods into our diet, including fruits, vegetables, whole grains, lean proteins, and healthy fats. By fueling our bodies with the right nutrients, we can maintain a healthy weight and support our overall health and well-being.

In conclusion, nourishing from within is essential for our physical and mental health. Understanding the importance of nutrition and making conscious choices about what we eat can lead to a healthier, happier, and more fulfilling life. So let's make nutrition a priority and give our body the proper fuel it needs to thrive. Let's choose food that nourishes us from within and empowers us to live our best life.

Chapter 3: The Power of Movement: How Exercise Benefits Our Physical and Mental Health

Introduction: We live in a fast-paced world where we are constantly bombarded with pressures and demands from all aspects of our lives. As a result, we often neglect our physical and mental well-being, which leads to a variety of health issues. However, incorporating regular exercise into our daily routine can have a profound impact on our overall health and well-being. In this chapter, we will explore the power of movement and how exercise can benefit our physical and mental health.

Physical Benefits of Exercise:

1. Improved Cardiovascular Health: The heart is an essential organ in the body that pumps blood and supplies oxygen to the rest of the body. Regular exercise, such as running, swimming, or biking, strengthens the heart muscles and improves its efficiency. This, in turn, reduces the risk of heart diseases such as heart attacks, strokes, and high blood pressure.

2. Weight Management: Exercise plays a crucial role in maintaining a healthy weight and preventing obesity. When we engage in physical activity, our

bodies burn calories, which helps to maintain a healthy balance between the calories we consume and the energy we expend. This is especially important in today's sedentary lifestyle where most of us spend long hours sitting at our desks.

3. Stronger Muscles and Bones: Resistance training, such as lifting weights, can increase muscle mass and improve bone density. This is particularly important as we age, as it helps to prevent conditions such as osteoporosis and sarcopenia, which can lead to weak bones and muscles.

4. Increased Flexibility and Balance: Regular exercise can improve flexibility and balance, which are essential for daily activities and preventing injuries. Activities such as yoga and Pilates can improve balance and flexibility, leading to better posture and reduced risk of falls in older adults.

5. Boosted Immune System: Exercise has been shown to improve the body's immune system, making us less susceptible to illnesses and infections. This is because physical activity increases the production of antibodies and white blood cells, which are crucial for fighting off infections and diseases.

Mental Benefits of Exercise:

1. Stress Relief: Exercise is a natural stress reliever as it helps to release endorphins, also known as "feel-good" hormones. These hormones improve our mood and help us feel more relaxed and at ease. This is particularly beneficial in today's high-stress society.

2. Improved Cognitive Function: Regular physical activity has been linked to improved cognitive function and a reduced risk of cognitive decline and dementia. This is because exercise increases blood flow to the brain, delivering essential oxygen and nutrients that help keep our brains healthy and functioning optimally.

3. Better Sleep: Exercise can help improve the quality of our sleep, leading to better rest and increased energy levels throughout the day. This is because physical activity helps to regulate our circadian rhythm, the body's natural sleep and wake cycle.

4. Increased Confidence and Self-Esteem: Engaging in regular exercise can also boost our confidence and self-esteem. As we see improvements in our physical health, we feel more confident in our

abilities and ourselves, leading to a more positive self-image.

5. Social Connection: Exercise can also provide an opportunity to connect with others, whether through group fitness classes or team sports. This social interaction can help reduce feelings of loneliness and improve our overall well-being.

Conclusion:

Regular exercise has numerous physical and mental health benefits that cannot be ignored. By incorporating some form of physical activity into our daily routine, we can improve our cardiovascular health, manage our weight, increase muscle and bone strength, and boost our immune system. Exercise also has significant mental health benefits, including stress relief, improved cognitive function, better sleep, increased confidence, and social connection. It is never too late to start reaping these benefits and making exercise a part of our lives. So, get moving and experience the power of movement for yourself!

Chapter 4: Finding Balance: Managing Stress and Prioritizing Self-Care

In today's fast-paced world, it can be easy to get caught up in the constant cycle of work and responsibilities. As a result, stress and burnout have become all too common among individuals of all ages and backgrounds. However, it is important to prioritize self-care and find balance in order to maintain our overall well-being.

What is stress?

Stress is our body's natural response to any demand or threat. It is a normal part of life and can be both positive and negative. Positive stress, or eustress, can motivate us and help us accomplish our goals and tasks. Negative stress, or distress, can cause harm to our physical and mental health if not managed properly.

Stress can manifest in various ways, such as headaches, muscle tension, fatigue, irritability, and changes in appetite or sleep patterns. If left unchecked, chronic stress can lead to more serious issues like anxiety, depression, and heart disease.

Why is self-care important?

Self-care refers to any deliberate actions we take to care for our physical, mental, and emotional well-being. It is vital for maintaining balance in our lives and managing stress effectively. Just like how we make time to take care of our responsibilities, it is equally important to make time for self-care. By prioritizing self-care, we can prevent burnout and improve our overall quality of life.

Tips for Managing Stress and Prioritizing Self-Care

1. Identify and Address Sources of Stress
The first step in managing stress is to identify what is causing it. Often, the root of stress lies in our daily responsibilities and expectations. Reflect on things that cause you the most stress and find ways to address or minimize them. This could mean delegating tasks, setting boundaries, or even saying "no" when necessary.

2. Practice Mindfulness
Mindfulness is the practice of being fully present in the moment without judging or reacting to our thoughts and emotions. It can help us become more aware of our stress triggers and learn to let go of negative thoughts and feelings. Incorporate mindfulness into your daily routine through

activities like meditation, breathing exercises, or simply taking a few moments to pause and focus on your surroundings.

3. Engage in Self-Care Activities
Self-care looks different for everyone, but the key is to engage in activities that bring you joy and help you relax. This could be anything from going for a walk in nature, reading a book, taking a bubble bath, or spending time with loved ones. Make a list of activities that make you feel good, and make an effort to incorporate at least one of them into your daily routine.

4. Prioritize Sleep and Nutrition
Getting enough sleep and eating a nutritious diet are essential for our overall well-being. Lack of sleep and poor nutrition can worsen stress and impact our physical health. Aim for 7-9 hours of sleep each night and prioritize whole, nutritious foods in your diet. This will give your body the fuel and rest it needs to manage stress effectively.

5. Set Realistic Goals and Prioritize Tasks
Often, we are our own worst critics, and we can put immense pressure on ourselves to accomplish everything on our to-do list. However, this can lead to overwhelm and burnout. Instead, set realistic goals and prioritize tasks based on their importance

and urgency. This will help you focus on what truly needs your attention and relieve the stress of trying to do everything at once.

Conclusion

In order to manage stress and find balance in our lives, it is crucial to prioritize self-care. By identifying sources of stress, practicing mindfulness, engaging in self-care activities, prioritizing sleep and nutrition, and setting realistic goals, we can effectively manage stress and improve our overall well-being. Remember to make self-care a priority and give yourself the time and space you need to maintain a healthy, balanced life.

Chapter 5: Healing from the Inside Out: The Role of Holistic and Alternative Medicine

In our society, we often turn to prescription medications as the go-to solution for any health issue. However, there has been a shift towards incorporating holistic and alternative medicine in recent years. This approach looks at the person as a whole, addressing not just physical symptoms but also emotional, mental, and spiritual well-being. In this chapter, we will explore the role of holistic and alternative medicine in healing from the inside out.

Holistic medicine takes into account all aspects of a person, including their lifestyle, diet, exercise, and stress levels. It believes that all of these factors play a crucial role in maintaining and restoring overall health. One of the key principles of holistic medicine is that the body has an innate ability to heal itself, and by addressing the root causes of illness, we can support this natural healing process.

Alternative medicine refers to a diverse range of therapies and practices that are not traditionally used in Western medicine. These include acupuncture, herbal remedies, homeopathy, energy healing, and many others. While some may view these practices as unproven or even controversial, many people have found great success in using them to treat a variety of health issues.

One of the main benefits of holistic and alternative medicine is its focus on prevention. Rather than waiting until a person is sick, these approaches prioritize maintaining overall health and preventing illness from occurring in the first place. This is done through techniques such as stress reduction, proper nutrition, and regular exercise. By taking care of the whole person, we can boost the immune system and reduce the risk of developing chronic diseases.

Another important aspect of holistic and alternative medicine is the emphasis on treating not just the physical symptoms of a disease, but also the underlying emotional and mental aspects. It is well-known that stress and other negative emotions can have a significant impact on our physical health, and addressing these issues can be crucial in achieving true healing. Alternative practices such as meditation, yoga, and mindfulness have been shown to reduce stress and improve overall well-being.

There is also a growing body of research that supports the use of alternative therapies in conjunction with conventional medicine. In some cases, these practices can help to reduce the dosage of medications needed or even replace them entirely. For example, acupuncture has been shown to be effective in managing pain, and in some cases, can be used as an alternative to pain medication. By incorporating alternative therapies into treatment plans, individuals can experience a more comprehensive and personalized approach to healing.

At its core, holistic and alternative medicine aims to treat the person, not just the disease. By considering all aspects of a person's life, including their physical, emotional, and spiritual well-being, we can promote healing from the inside out. This approach can be used to address a wide range of health issues, from chronic pain to mental health disorders to autoimmune diseases.

For those who may be skeptical of these practices, it is important to note that they are not meant to replace traditional medicine. Instead, they can be used in conjunction with conventional treatments to enhance overall health and well-being. As with any medical treatment, it is essential to consult with a licensed practitioner before starting any new therapy.

In conclusion, holistic and alternative medicine offer a unique and valuable approach to healing from the inside out. By considering the whole person and utilizing a variety of practices and therapies, individuals can achieve optimal health and well-being. As we continue to learn more about the interconnectedness of mind, body, and spirit, it is becoming increasingly clear that addressing all of these aspects is crucial for long-term health and healing.

Chapter 6: The Importance of Sleep: How Quality Rest Can Transform Your Health

In today's fast-paced and busy world, sleep is often seen as a luxury rather than a necessity. Many people view it as a waste of time and prioritize other activities such as work, socializing, or hobbies. However, the truth is that quality sleep is essential for our overall health and well-being.

As humans, we spend approximately one-third of our lives sleeping. This may seem like a large chunk of time, but the importance of sleep cannot be overstated. It is during this restful state that our body repairs and rejuvenates itself, allowing us to function at our best during our waking hours.

So, what exactly is quality sleep, and why is it important? Quality sleep refers to getting enough hours of uninterrupted, deep, and restorative sleep. It involves going through different stages of sleep, including light sleep, deep sleep, and REM (rapid eye movement) sleep. Each stage plays a crucial role in maintaining our physical, mental, and emotional well-being.

Now, let's dive into the benefits of quality sleep and why it is worth prioritizing in our daily lives.

1. Boosts physical health:

Quality sleep is essential for our physical health, as it allows our body to repair and heal itself. During sleep, the body releases growth hormones that repair damaged cells, tissues, and muscles. Inadequate sleep can lead to a weakened immune system, making us more susceptible to illnesses and infections.

Moreover, good sleep also plays a significant role in maintaining a healthy weight. Lack of sleep has been linked to an increase in appetite and a decrease in the hormone leptin, which signals the body when we are full. This can lead to overeating and weight gain.

2. Sharpens Cognitive Functioning:

Sleep is crucial for our brain's optimal functioning. It allows our brain to rest, recharge, and consolidate memories, which are essential for learning and retaining information. Quality sleep has also been linked to better concentration, problem-solving skills, and creativity.

On the other hand, lack of sleep can result in fatigue, decreased alertness, and impaired cognitive functioning. This can lead to poor judgment, increased risk of accidents, and decreased productivity.

3. Improves Mental Health:

Getting enough quality sleep is vital for our emotional and mental well-being. Adequate sleep helps regulate our mood and emotions, making us less irritable and more emotionally stable. On the other hand, a lack of sleep has been linked to increased levels of the stress hormone cortisol, which can contribute to anxiety and depression.

4. Promotes Healthy Aging:

Quality sleep is essential for anti-aging and promoting longevity. During sleep, our body produces a hormone called melatonin, which acts as an antioxidant, protecting our cells from damage. It also promotes the production of collagen, essential for maintaining healthy skin and preventing premature aging.

Moreover, lack of sleep has been linked to a higher risk of chronic diseases such as heart disease, diabetes, and obesity, affecting the aging process and overall health.

So, how can we ensure we get enough quality sleep? Here are some tips:

1. Stick to a consistent sleep schedule: Try to go to bed and wake up at the same time every day, even on weekends.

2. Create a comfortable sleep environment: Make sure your room is dark, quiet, and cool to optimize your sleep quality.

3. Limit screen time before bed: Electronics emit blue light, which suppresses melatonin production and affects our sleep-wake cycle. Avoid using screens at least an hour before bedtime.

4. Limit caffeine and alcohol: Avoid consuming caffeine and alcohol close to bedtime, as they can interfere with sleep patterns.

5. Practice relaxation techniques: Taking a warm bath, meditating, or practicing deep breathing exercises can help relax your body and mind for better sleep.

In conclusion sleep is not a waste of time, but a crucial aspect of our overall and well-being. Prioritizing and consistently getting enough quality sleep can have a transformative effect on our physical, mental, and emotional health. So, make sure to give yourself the gift of a good night's rest and reap the numerous benefits it has to offer.

Chapter 7: Cultivating Healthy Relationships: The Impact of Social Connections on Our Well-Being

As human beings, we are inherently social creatures. We crave connection and interaction with others, and our relationships with those around us greatly impact our overall well-being. Healthy relationships are essential for our emotional, mental, and even physical health. In this chapter, we will delve into the importance of cultivating healthy relationships and how they impact our lives.

The Power of Social Connection
Social connection is the bond we feel with others, whether it be with family, friends, romantic partners, or even our community as a whole. This connection is vital for our survival and has been shown to have profound effects on our health and well-being.

Studies have shown that those with strong social connections have a lower risk of mental health issues such as depression and anxiety. This is because social interaction can provide a sense of support, belonging, and purpose. Feeling connected to others also leads to higher self-esteem and a more positive outlook on life.

Additionally, social connection has been linked to physical health. People with strong social ties have a lower risk of developing chronic illnesses such as heart disease, high blood pressure, and even cancer. The support and love we receive from our social connections can help us cope with stress and boost our immune system.

Benefits of Healthy Relationships
Now that we understand the impact of social connections, let's explore the benefits of cultivating healthy relationships. A healthy relationship is characterized by trust, respect, communication, and support. It is a two-way street where both parties contribute to the well-being of the relationship.

One of the main benefits of a healthy relationship is increased happiness. When we feel loved, supported, and understood by those around us, we are more content and fulfilled in our lives. This, in turn, leads to a more positive outlook and increased life satisfaction.

A healthy relationship can also enhance our personal growth and development. Through our interactions with others, we learn more about ourselves, our values, and how to communicate effectively. We can also learn from the different perspectives and experiences of those in our social circle, allowing us to broaden our horizons and become more empathetic and understanding individuals.

Finally, healthy relationships can also provide a support system during times of stress and hardship. Whether it be a shoulder to cry on, a listening ear, or practical assistance, having strong relationships can help us navigate through difficult times and come out stronger on the other side.

Nurturing Healthy Relationships
So how do we cultivate healthy relationships in our lives? The key is to be intentional and proactive in our relationships. Take the time to nurture and maintain the connections you have with others. Here are some ways to do so:

1. Communication: Good communication is essential for any relationship. Be open, honest, and respectful when expressing yourself, and actively listen to others.

2. Boundaries: Establishing boundaries is crucial to maintaining a healthy relationship. This involves knowing your limits, respecting the boundaries of others, and speaking up when those boundaries are crossed.

3. Quality time: Set aside time to spend with your loved ones without distractions such as phones or TV. This dedicated time allows for deeper and more meaningful connections.

4. Support: Be there for your loved ones during both the good and bad times. Offer your support, whether it be emotional or practical, and accept support when it is offered to you.

5. Appreciation: Show your appreciation for your loved ones. A simple 'thank you' or token of gratitude can go a long way in strengthening a relationship.

6. Conflict resolution: Conflicts are bound to happen in any relationship, but it is how we handle them that matters. Communicate calmly and work towards finding a resolution that is mutually beneficial.

In conclusion, healthy relationships are vital for our overall well-being. They provide us with a sense of belonging, support, personal growth, and happiness. By being intentional and proactive and cultivating healthy relationships, we can reap the many benefits they offer. So take the time to nurture your relationships and watch how they positively impact your life.

Chapter 8: The Science of Happiness: How Positive Emotions Can Lead to Optimal Health

As human beings, we all have an innate desire to be happy. It is a universal goal that transcends cultural, social, and economic boundaries. But what exactly is happiness? This elusive concept has been studied and contemplated by philosophers, psychologists, and scientists for centuries. It is a complex and multifaceted emotion that can be difficult to define and measure. However, in recent years, there has been a growing body of research that sheds light on the science of happiness and its impact on our overall wellbeing.

Happiness is a positive psychological state that encompasses feelings of joy, contentment, and fulfillment. It is not a constant state but rather a fluctuating emotion that can be influenced by various internal and external factors. While some people may have a naturally optimistic disposition, studies have shown that happiness is, to a large extent, within our control. This means that we have the ability to cultivate and maintain positive emotions, which can have a significant impact on our physical, mental, and emotional health.

One of the key components of the science of happiness is the concept of positive emotions. These include love, joy, gratitude, hope, contentment, and many others. Positive emotions have been described as fleeting feelings of pleasure that are often associated with specific events or experiences. For example, the feeling of joy when receiving a promotion or the sense of awe and wonder while watching a beautiful sunset. These emotions have been linked to several physical and psychological benefits that can promote overall wellbeing.

One of the most significant ways that positive emotions can benefit our health is through their influence on the autonomic nervous system. This system is responsible for regulating several bodily functions, including heart rate, blood pressure, and digestion. Research has shown that positive emotions can increase parasympathetic activity, which is responsible for relaxation, and decrease sympathetic activity, which is associated with stress responses. This can lead to lower levels of stress hormones and improved immune function, ultimately reducing the risk of several chronic diseases.

Furthermore, studies have shown that positive emotions can lead to a better quality of life. People who experience positive emotions regularly are more satisfied with life, have higher self-esteem, and report better social relationships. This is because positive emotions have been found to increase feelings of connectedness and strengthen social bonds. As social creatures, humans thrive on positive social interactions, and these emotions can act as a powerful social lubricant.

In addition to physiological and social benefits, positive emotions can also have a significant impact on our mental health. Multiple studies have found a strong correlation between positive emotions and decreased symptoms of depression and anxiety. This is because positive emotions can promote a sense of resilience and optimism, which can help individuals cope with negative experiences and emotions effectively. Just as negative emotions can contribute to mental health issues, positive emotions can act as a protective factor against them.

So, how can we cultivate and increase positive emotions in our daily lives? The good news is that there are several evidence-based practices that have been shown to have a positive impact on mood and wellbeing. Expressing gratitude, practicing mindfulness, and participating in activities that bring joy and pleasure are just a few examples. Additionally, engaging in acts of kindness and cultivating positive relationships can also boost positive emotions. These practices may seem simple, but incorporating them into our daily routines can have a significant impact on our overall happiness and health.

In conclusion, the science of happiness teaches us that positive emotions can have a profound impact on our physical, mental, and emotional wellbeing. By understanding and utilizing this knowledge, we can take control of our happiness and lead a healthier and more fulfilling life. So, make a conscious effort to cultivate positive emotions, and watch as they contribute to your overall happiness and optimal health.

Chapter 9: Unlocking Your Inner Potential: Strategies for Personal Growth and Development

We all have infinite potential within us, waiting to be unlocked and harnessed. However, many of us often let fear, self-doubt, and limiting beliefs hold us back from reaching our full potential. But the truth is, when we tap into our inner potential, we can achieve anything we set our minds to.

In this chapter, we will explore various strategies for personal growth and development that will help you unlock your inner potential and become the best version of yourself.

1. Know Yourself

The first step towards unlocking your inner potential is to truly know yourself—your strengths, weaknesses, values, and aspirations. Take time to reflect on your past experiences, your accomplishments, and your failures. Identify your skills and talents, and also acknowledge your areas for improvement. This self-awareness will provide you with a solid foundation to work on and develop yourself.

2. Set Goals

Once you have a good understanding of yourself, it's time to set some goals. Goals give you direction and something to strive for. They should be specific, measurable, achievable, relevant, and time-bound (SMART) to increase your chances of success. Additionally, make sure your goals align with your values and purpose, as this will give you the motivation and determination to achieve them.

3. Continuously Learn and Grow

Learning should not stop after you finish your formal education. To unlock your inner potential, you must be open to continuous learning and growth. This can be in the form of taking a class, attending a workshop, reading books, or even gaining new experiences. Each new skill or piece of knowledge you acquire will contribute to your personal growth and development.

4. Step Out of Your Comfort Zone

We often think and act within our comfort zones because it feels safe and familiar. However, real growth and development happen when we step out of our comfort zones. It's where we push our limits, face our fears, and discover our true potential. So challenge yourself to try new things, take risks, and embrace change. You never know what you are capable of until you try.

5. Cultivate a Growth Mindset

Having a growth mindset means believing that your abilities can be developed through hard work, dedication, and persistence. On the other hand, a fixed mindset believes that talents and traits are fixed and cannot be changed. To unlock your inner potential, you must cultivate a growth mindset. This will help you approach challenges and setbacks as opportunities to learn and improve, rather than viewing them as failures.

6. Surround Yourself with Positive and Supportive People

The people we surround ourselves with can greatly influence our thoughts, behaviors, and attitudes. Therefore, it's essential to surround ourselves with positive and supportive people who believe in us and our potential. These individuals will encourage and motivate us to become our best selves, and their positive energy will make a significant impact on our personal growth and development.

7. Practice Self-Care and Self-Compassion

Taking care of ourselves is crucial for our well-being and personal growth. We must prioritize self-care by getting enough rest, eating well, and engaging in activities that bring us joy and relaxation. Along with self-care, self-compassion is also essential. We must learn to be kind to ourselves and practice self-acceptance, especially during times of failure or setbacks. Self-compassion allows us to bounce back stronger and continue our journey towards unlocking our inner potential.

8. Embrace Failure and Learn from it

Failure is a natural part of life, and it's important to embrace it as a learning opportunity. When we fail, we must take the time to reflect on what went wrong and what we can do better next time. Instead of dwelling on our failures, we must use them as stepping stones towards growth and improvement.

In conclusion, unlocking your inner potential is a continuous journey of self-discovery and growth. By knowing yourself, setting goals, learning and growing, stepping out of your comfort zone, cultivating a growth mindset, surrounding yourself with positive people, practicing self-care and compassion, and embracing failure, you can tap into your limitless potential and become the best version of yourself. So go out there and unlock your inner potential – the possibilities are endless!

Chapter 10: From Surviving to Thriving: Creating a Sustainable and Fulfilling Lifestyle

In today's fast-paced and consumer-driven world, it's easy to get caught up in the rat race of simply surviving. Many people find themselves working long hours and sacrificing personal well-being for the sake of financial stability and success. However, what many fail to realize is that this constant cycle of survival is not sustainable and can lead to physical, mental, and emotional exhaustion.

It's time to shift our focus from just surviving to thriving. In this chapter, I will share with you the key components of creating a sustainable and fulfilling lifestyle that will not only improve your overall well-being but also set you up for long-term success and happiness.

1. Identify Your Values and Priorities:
The first step in creating a sustainable and fulfilling lifestyle is to identify your core values and priorities. These are the things that truly matter to you and define who you are as a person. Take some time to reflect on what aspects of life bring you the most joy and fulfillment, whether it's family, friends, career, personal growth, or leisure activities. Once you have a clear understanding of

your values and priorities, you can align your actions and decisions with them, leading to a more fulfilling and purposeful life.

2. Practice mindfulness:
Mindfulness is the practice of being present and fully engaged in the current moment. In our fast-paced world, it's easy to get caught up in the endless stream of thoughts and distractions. By practicing mindfulness, you can quiet your mind and focus on the present, which can reduce stress and increase overall well-being. This can be done through activities such as meditation, yoga, and mindful breathing exercises.

3. Create a Healthy Work-Life Balance:
One of the most common reasons for burnout and exhaustion is an imbalance between work and personal life. It's essential to establish boundaries and prioritize self-care to avoid being consumed by work. Set aside time for activities that bring you joy and rejuvenate your mind, body, and soul. This can include hobbies, spending time with loved ones, and taking breaks from work to recharge.

4. Pursue Meaningful Relationships:
Humans are social beings, and meaningful connections with others can bring immense fulfillment and happiness. Take the time to cultivate

and nurture genuine relationships with friends, family, and a significant other. Make an effort to communicate openly and listen to others without judgment. When you have a strong support system, you can face challenges more confidently and share in life's joys and successes.

5. Invest in Personal Growth:
Continuous personal growth is vital for a sustainable and fulfilling lifestyle. This can involve learning new skills, taking on new challenges, and stepping out of your comfort zone. Set personal goals and work towards them, whether it's in your career or personal life. When you invest in your personal growth, you will not only achieve a sense of accomplishment but also gain a deeper understanding of yourself.

6. Prioritize Physical and Mental Health:
A sustainable and fulfilling lifestyle requires a healthy mind and body. Take care of your physical health by getting regular exercise, eating a balanced and nutritious diet, and getting enough rest. Prioritizing your mental health is just as crucial. Seek professional support if necessary, and practice self-care activities such as journaling, spending time in nature, and engaging in hobbies you enjoy.

In conclusion, creating a sustainable and fulfilling lifestyle is a continuous process. It requires reflection, intention, and consistent effort to align your actions with your values and priorities. By incorporating these key components into your life, you can move from simply surviving to thriving and lead a fulfilling and purposeful life.

Conclusion: Embracing Your Journey to Optimal Health

Congratulations, dear reader! You have made it to the end of this book, and I hope that throughout your reading journey, you have gained valuable insights and knowledge on how to achieve optimal health. I want to take this opportunity to thank you for joining me on this journey, and I truly hope that you have found this book to be informative, inspiring, and empowering.

Now, at this point, you might be wondering, "What exactly is optimal health? And how can I achieve it?" Well, these are great questions, and the answers to them are what this book is all about.

Optimal health can be defined as a state of physical, mental, and social well-being, not just the absence of disease or infirmity. It is about feeling your best, both physically and mentally, and being able to live your life to the fullest. Optimal health is not a destination; it is a journey that requires dedication, commitment, and a willingness to continually learn and adapt.

In this book, we have covered various aspects of optimal health, including nutrition, exercise, stress management, and self-care. We have discussed the importance of nourishing our bodies with whole and nutrient-dense foods and how proper nutrition can impact our physical and mental well-being. We have also explored different types of exercise and how regular physical activity can improve our overall health and quality of life.

Additionally, we have delved into the topic of stress and how it affects our bodies and minds. Through various techniques and tips, we have learned how to manage stress effectively and develop a more peaceful and balanced life.

One crucial aspect of optimal health that we have discussed is self-care. It is essential to prioritize ourselves and our well-being, and self-care is a vital part of this. It is about taking the time to do things that bring us joy, peace, and balance. Whether it is reading a book, taking a bath, or going for a walk, self-care should be a non-negotiable part of our daily routine.

I want to emphasize that achieving optimal health is not a one-size-fits-all approach. What works for one individual may not work for another, and that is okay. It is essential to listen to your body and find what nourishes and supports you the most. It is also essential to remember that optimal health is a continuous journey, and it requires constant effort and evaluation.

As I mentioned earlier, this book is not just about physical health. It is also about mental and social well-being. Mental health is just as important as physical health, and it should not be ignored. Taking care of our minds is crucial for our overall well-being. It is okay to seek help and support when needed, and there should be no shame or stigma attached to that.

Lastly, I want to encourage you to embrace your journey to optimal health. It is not always easy, and there will be ups and downs, but the key is to keep going and never give up. Always remember that you are worth the effort, and your health and well-being should always be a priority.

Thank you again for joining me on this journey, and I wish you all the best on your path to optimal health. Remember to be kind to yourself, listen to your body, and enjoy the process. Cheers to a happy and healthy life!